# Why Smoking?

# Want to stop Smoking!

# Content

Chapter 1: Lighting the Way: Understanding the Smoking Trap

- This chapter explores the psychology behind smoking, examining the addictive nature of nicotine and the various factors that contribute to the smoking habit. It delves into the physical, emotional, and social aspects of smoking, helping readers gain a deeper understanding of why they smoke.

Chapter 2: Clearing the Air: Unveiling the Health Risks

- In this chapter, the focus shifts to the detrimental health effects of smoking. It provides comprehensive information on the various diseases and conditions associated with smoking, including lung cancer, heart disease, and respiratory disorders. The chapter emphasizes the importance of prioritizing one's health and the benefits of quitting smoking.

Chapter 3: Breaking the Chains: Strategies for Overcoming Addiction

- This chapter explores effective strategies and techniques for quitting smoking. It discusses nicotine replacement therapy, medications, behavioral therapies, and support systems that can aid in the journey towards quitting. It also provides tips on managing cravings, coping with withdrawal symptoms, and staying motivated throughout the quitting process.

Chapter 4: Rewriting the Narrative: Changing Your Mindset

- Shifting the focus to the power of the mind, this chapter delves into the importance of changing one's mindset and beliefs about smoking. It explores the role of self-talk, visualization, and positive affirmations in overcoming addiction. Readers are guided on reframing their thoughts, building resilience, and adopting a new, smoke-free identity.

Chapter 5: Smoke-Free Living: Creating Healthy Habits

- This chapter provides practical guidance on creating a smoke-free environment and adopting healthier habits. It covers topics such as managing triggers and temptations, finding alternative coping mechanisms, incorporating exercise and mindfulness into daily routines, and building a support network of non-smoking individuals.

Chapter 6: Nurturing the Smoke-Free You: Self-Care and Wellbeing

- Focusing on self-care and holistic wellbeing, this chapter emphasizes the importance of nurturing oneself during the quitting process. It explores self-care practices, stress management techniques, and strategies for boosting mental and emotional resilience. The chapter also highlights the rewards and positive changes that come with a smoke-free lifestyle.

Chapter 7: Embracing the Smoke-Free Future: Sustaining Success

- In the final chapter, readers are encouraged to celebrate their achievements and plan for a sustainable smoke-free future. It provides guidance on preventing relapse, managing potential setbacks, and staying committed to a healthy, smoke-free life. The chapter also emphasizes the long-term benefits of quitting smoking and the positive impact it has on one's overall wellbeing.

# Chapter 1: Lighting the Way: Understanding the Smoking Trap

Introduction:

Smoking—a seemingly innocuous act that holds millions of people in its clutches. It begins with a puff, a taste, a momentary escape from reality. But little do we know, it sets in motion a cycle of addiction that can consume us for years, if not decades. In this chapter, we embark on a journey to unravel the enigma of smoking, peering into the depths of its allure and understanding the complex web it weaves in our lives.

## Section 1: The Nicotine Connection

We dive straight into the heart of the matter: nicotine—the driving force behind the smoking trap. Exploring the science of addiction, we delve into the intricate mechanisms by which nicotine hijacks our brain and fuels the craving for more. We examine the role of dopamine, the brain's reward system, and how it becomes entangled in the grip of nicotine.

## Section 2: The Smoking Habit

Here, we turn our attention to the behavioral patterns and habits that intertwine with smoking.

From the rituals surrounding lighting up to the associations with certain activities or social settings, we dissect the multifaceted nature of the smoking habit. We delve into the psychology of smoking and the emotional triggers that compel individuals to reach for a cigarette.

Section 3: Social Pressures and Smoking

No discussion about smoking is complete without acknowledging the social factors that contribute to its prevalence. Peer influence, societal norms, and the portrayal of smoking in media all play a significant role in perpetuating the habit. We examine the impact of advertising, cultural factors, and the power of social connections in shaping our smoking behavior.

Section 4: Escaping the Smoke Screen: The Motivations to Quit

In this section, we explore the various motivations that lead individuals to contemplate quitting smoking. From health concerns to financial burdens, we uncover the compelling reasons why people embark on the journey to become smoke-free. By understanding these motivations, readers can gain clarity on their own desires and find the inner strength to break free.

Section 5: The Cycle of Relapse

Quitting smoking is a battle fraught with challenges, and understanding the cycle of relapse is essential to overcoming them. We examine the common pitfalls that can derail even the most determined quitters. From the allure of "just one more cigarette" to the triggers that can reignite the smoking habit, we shed light on the obstacles that lie in wait.

Conclusion:

As we conclude this chapter, we have scratched the surface of the smoking trap, peering into the complexities that keep individuals bound to the habit. Armed with knowledge, we are better equipped to understand our own relationship with smoking and lay the foundation for a journey towards freedom. The path ahead may be challenging, but with each step, we inch closer to a life liberated from the clutches of smoke.

# Chapter 2: Clearing the Air: Unveiling the Health Risks

Introduction:

While the allure of smoking may seem enticing, it is crucial to confront the harsh reality of its impact on our health. In this chapter, we delve into the dark side of smoking, shining a light on the numerous health risks associated with this harmful habit. By understanding the toll smoking takes on our bodies, we can find the motivation to prioritize our well-being and break free from the grip of tobacco.

## Section 1: The Lungs: Targets of Destruction

We begin by exploring the devastating effects smoking has on our lungs. From chronic bronchitis to emphysema, we unravel the intricate web of respiratory diseases that can manifest as a result of smoking. Through vivid descriptions and medical insights, we paint a vivid picture of the gradual deterioration that occurs within the lungs of smokers.

## Section 2: Heart and Circulatory System: A Looming Danger

In this section, we turn our attention to the cardiovascular system, revealing the hidden dangers smoking poses to our heart and blood vessels. We delve into the heightened risk of heart disease, hypertension, and stroke that accompanies the smoking habit. By understanding the mechanisms behind these conditions, readers can grasp the urgency of quitting smoking for the sake of their cardiovascular health.

Section 3: Beyond the Lungs and Heart: A Comprehensive Look at Smoking-Related Diseases

Smoking's detrimental effects are not confined to the respiratory and cardiovascular systems alone. In this section, we broaden our scope to explore the wider range of diseases linked to smoking. From various types of cancer, including lung, throat, and bladder cancer, to the increased susceptibility to infections and compromised immune function, we shine a light on the comprehensive impact smoking has on our overall health.

Section 4: Secondhand Smoke: A Silent Threat

Smoking doesn't just harm the individuals who light up—it poses risks to those around them as well. We examine the concept of secondhand smoke and the dangers it presents to nonsmokers, particularly vulnerable populations such as children and pregnant women. By shedding light on the effects of secondhand smoke, we inspire readers to consider the impact their smoking has on loved ones and acquaintances.

Section 5: The Price of Smoking: Financial and Social Costs

Beyond the toll it takes on our health, smoking exacts a significant financial and social burden. We explore the economic consequences of smoking, including the costs of purchasing cigarettes, healthcare expenses, and lost productivity. Furthermore, we delve into the social implications, such as the stigma associated with smoking and the potential strain it puts on relationships.

Conclusion:

As we conclude this chapter, the fog of ignorance surrounding the health risks of smoking has begun to dissipate. We have exposed the toll it takes on our lungs, heart, and overall well-being. Armed with this knowledge, we can no longer turn a blind eye to the consequences of smoking. It is time to take charge of our health, prioritize our well-being, and embrace a smoke-free future.

# Chapter 3: Breaking the Chains: Strategies for Overcoming Addiction

Introduction:

Now that we have gained an understanding of the allure of smoking and the health risks it poses, it is time to equip ourselves with the tools necessary to break free from this addictive habit. In this chapter, we explore a range of effective strategies and techniques designed to help individuals overcome their addiction to smoking. By implementing these strategies, readers can embark on a journey towards a healthier, smoke-free life.

## Section 1: Nicotine Replacement Therapy: A Path to Liberation

One approach to quitting smoking is through nicotine replacement therapy (NRT). We delve into the various NRT options available, such as nicotine gum, patches, nasal sprays, inhalers, and lozenges. By understanding how NRT works and its potential benefits, readers can make informed decisions about incorporating these aids into their quit-smoking journey.

Section 2: Medications to Aid in Quitting

In this section, we explore medications that can assist individuals in their quest to quit smoking. We delve into the efficacy and potential side effects of prescription medications, such as varenicline and bupropion. By understanding how these medications work and consulting with healthcare professionals, readers can determine if medication-assisted quitting is a suitable option for them.

Section 3: Behavioral Therapies: Rewiring the Mind

Breaking the cycle of addiction requires addressing the behavioral patterns associated with smoking. We examine various behavioral therapies, such as cognitive-behavioral therapy (CBT), motivational interviewing, and mindfulness-based techniques. By incorporating these therapies into their quit-smoking journey, readers can gain insights into their triggers, develop coping mechanisms, and reshape their relationship with smoking.

Section 4: Support Systems: Strength in Numbers

Quitting smoking can be a challenging endeavor, but it becomes more manageable with the support of others. We discuss the importance of support systems, including family, friends, and support groups. We explore resources such as smoking cessation helplines, online communities, and counseling services, offering readers the tools to build a strong support network that will bolster their efforts to quit smoking.

Section 5: Managing Cravings and Withdrawal Symptoms

Cravings and withdrawal symptoms can pose significant obstacles to quitting smoking. In this section, we provide practical tips and techniques to manage cravings effectively. From distraction techniques and deep breathing exercises to engaging in physical activities and adopting healthy coping mechanisms, readers will discover an arsenal of strategies to navigate the challenging moments of withdrawal.

Section 6: Staying Motivated: Fostering Determination and Resilience

Quitting smoking is a journey that requires unwavering determination and resilience. We explore methods for staying motivated and maintaining focus on the goal of becoming smoke-free. We discuss the power of setting personal goals, celebrating milestones, and cultivating a positive mindset. By fostering determination and resilience, readers will be better equipped to navigate the ups and downs of the quitting process.

Conclusion:

As we conclude this chapter, readers are armed with a range of strategies and techniques to aid them in their quest to overcome addiction and quit smoking. By combining nicotine replacement therapy, medications, behavioral therapies, and support systems, individuals can increase their chances of success. Remember, the road to freedom from smoking may have its challenges, but with the right tools and support, a smoke-free life is well within reach.

# Chapter 4: Rewriting the Narrative: Changing Your Mindset

Introduction:

Breaking free from the grip of smoking requires more than just physical strategies; it necessitates a shift in mindset. In this chapter, we delve into the power of the mind and explore the importance of changing our beliefs, thoughts, and attitudes towards smoking. By rewiring our mindset, we can cultivate a smoke-free identity and pave the way for lasting change.

Section 1: The Power of Self-Talk: Shifting the Inner Dialogue

The words we speak to ourselves have a profound impact on our actions and behaviors. We explore the concept of self-talk and its influence on our smoking habits. By identifying and challenging negative self-talk related to smoking, readers can develop a more supportive and empowering internal dialogue that bolsters their motivation to quit.

## Section 2: Visualization Techniques: Seeing a Smoke-Free Future

Visualization is a powerful tool for manifesting change in our lives. We guide readers through visualization exercises specifically tailored to quitting smoking. By vividly imagining a smoke-free future and connecting with the positive emotions and benefits associated with it, readers can strengthen their resolve and reinforce their commitment to a life without cigarettes.

## Section 3: Affirmations: Harnessing the Power of Positive Declarations

Affirmations are positive statements that can reshape our thoughts and beliefs. We delve into the practice of using affirmations to reinforce a smoke-free mindset. By crafting personalized affirmations and incorporating them into daily routines, readers can replace limiting beliefs with empowering ones, bolstering their confidence and determination to overcome the smoking habit.

Section 4: Identifying and Managing Triggers: Taking Control of Smoking Associations

Triggers are situations, emotions, or activities that prompt the urge to smoke. We explore the common triggers associated with smoking and guide readers in identifying their personal triggers. By recognizing and understanding these triggers, readers can develop proactive strategies to manage them effectively, reducing the likelihood of relapse and empowering themselves to stay smoke-free.

Section 5: Reinventing Your Identity: Embracing the Smoke-Free You

Quitting smoking involves a transformation of identity—a shift from being a smoker to becoming a smoke-free individual. We explore techniques to help readers embrace this new identity and align their actions with their desired smoke-free self. By embracing a positive self-image and integrating smoke-free behaviors into their daily lives, readers can reinforce their commitment to long-term change.

Section 6: Building Resilience: Bouncing Back from Setbacks

The quitting journey may have its ups and downs, and resilience is key to maintaining progress. We explore strategies for building resilience and navigating potential setbacks or slip-ups. By cultivating a growth mindset, practicing self-compassion, and learning from challenges, readers can bounce back stronger and stay committed to their smoke-free goals.

Conclusion:

As we conclude this chapter, readers are equipped with the tools to rewrite the narrative surrounding smoking. By harnessing the power of self-talk, visualization, affirmations, and by identifying triggers and reinventing their identity, readers can create a mindset that supports a smoke-free life. With resilience as their foundation, they can overcome obstacles and stay committed to their journey of transformation. Remember, the power to break free from smoking lies within the power of your own mind.

# Chapter 5: Smoke-Free Living: Creating Healthy Habits

Introduction:

Quitting smoking is not just about eliminating a negative habit; it's about embracing a healthier lifestyle. In this chapter, we explore the importance of creating new, positive habits that support a smoke-free life. By replacing old routines and behaviors with healthier alternatives, readers can establish a foundation for long-term success and well-being.

## Section 1: Managing Triggers and Temptations

Successfully navigating triggers and temptations is crucial for maintaining a smoke-free lifestyle. We delve deeper into the strategies for managing common triggers, such as stress, social situations, and habitual routines. By identifying healthier coping mechanisms and developing alternative responses to triggers, readers can overcome challenges and reduce the urge to smoke.

## Section 2: Finding Alternative Coping Mechanisms

Smoking often serves as a coping mechanism for stress, boredom, or emotional turmoil. In this section, we explore a range of alternative coping mechanisms that can replace the habit of smoking. From engaging in physical activities and hobbies to practicing relaxation techniques and mindfulness, readers can discover healthier ways to manage their emotions and stress levels.

Section 3: Incorporating Exercise into Daily Life

Exercise not only promotes physical well-being but also plays a significant role in supporting a smoke-free life. We explore the benefits of regular physical activity and provide practical tips for incorporating exercise into daily routines. By embracing an active lifestyle, readers can experience increased energy, improved mood, and reduced cravings, fostering their commitment to staying smoke-free.

Section 4: Mindful Living: Cultivating Awareness and Presence

Mindfulness is a powerful practice that helps individuals develop greater awareness of their thoughts, emotions, and actions. We delve into the principles of mindfulness and its application in the context of quitting smoking. By cultivating present-moment awareness and mindfulness-based techniques, readers can develop a heightened sense of self-control, making it easier to resist the urge to smoke.

## Section 5: Nurturing Healthy Relationships and Social Connections

Healthy relationships and a supportive social network play a pivotal role in maintaining a smoke-free life. We explore the importance of nurturing positive relationships and seeking support from loved ones. Additionally, we discuss strategies for navigating social situations where smoking may be present, empowering readers to stay true to their smoke-free goals while fostering meaningful connections.

## Section 6: Reinventing Daily Rituals and Environments

Quitting smoking provides an opportunity to reinvent daily rituals and environments that were once associated with smoking. We delve into practical tips for transforming smoking-related habits and spaces into supportive, smoke-free environments. By redesigning routines, decluttering smoking paraphernalia, and creating new positive associations, readers can solidify their commitment to a smoke-free life.

Conclusion:

As we conclude this chapter, readers are encouraged to embrace a smoke-free lifestyle by creating healthy habits that support their long-term well-being. By effectively managing triggers and temptations, finding alternative coping mechanisms, incorporating exercise and mindfulness into daily routines, nurturing healthy relationships, and redesigning their environments, readers can establish a foundation for a fulfilling and smoke-free life. Remember, by prioritizing health and well-being, you are actively creating a brighter and healthier future for yourself.

# Chapter 6: Overcoming Challenges: Staying Strong in the Face of Obstacles

Introduction:

The journey to a smoke-free life is not without its challenges. In this chapter, we explore the common obstacles individuals may encounter on their path to quitting smoking and provide strategies for overcoming them. By understanding and proactively addressing these challenges, readers can fortify their resolve and stay strong in their commitment to living smoke-free.

## Section 1: Nicotine Withdrawal: Navigating the Initial Phase

Nicotine withdrawal can be one of the most challenging aspects of quitting smoking. We delve into the symptoms of withdrawal, both physical and psychological, and discuss strategies for managing them. By understanding the temporary nature of withdrawal symptoms and implementing coping mechanisms, readers can navigate this crucial phase of the quitting process.

## Section 2: Dealing with Cravings and Urges

Cravings and urges to smoke can be powerful triggers that test one's determination to quit. We explore practical techniques for managing and overcoming cravings. From distraction techniques and relaxation exercises to engaging in healthy habits and utilizing support systems, readers will gain valuable tools for conquering cravings and staying on track.

Section 3: Managing Stress and Emotional Triggers

Stress and emotional triggers can pose significant challenges during the quitting process. We delve into strategies for managing stress and effectively coping with emotions without relying on smoking. By exploring stress reduction techniques, developing emotional resilience, and seeking support, readers can develop healthier ways of managing stress and emotions.

Section 4: Dealing with Relapses: Learning from Setbacks

Relapses are common on the journey to quitting smoking, but they don't have to derail progress. We discuss the importance of viewing relapses as learning opportunities rather than failures. By understanding the triggers and circumstances that led to a relapse, readers can develop strategies to prevent future setbacks and strengthen their resolve to remain smoke-free.

## Section 5: Maintaining Motivation: Celebrating Milestones and Setting Goals

Sustaining motivation throughout the quitting process is essential for long-term success. We explore the power of celebrating milestones, setting new goals, and visualizing the benefits of a smoke-free life. By regularly acknowledging and rewarding progress, readers can stay motivated, reinforce their commitment, and continue to strive towards a healthier future.

## Section 6: Finding Meaning and Purpose Beyond Smoking

Quitting smoking opens up new opportunities for individuals to discover and pursue their passions. We delve into the process of finding meaning and purpose beyond smoking, exploring ways to cultivate a fulfilling life. By engaging in activities that align with personal values and aspirations, readers can create a sense of purpose that transcends the smoking habit.

Conclusion:

As we conclude this chapter, readers are armed with strategies for overcoming challenges and staying strong in their quest for a smoke-free life. By navigating nicotine withdrawal, managing cravings and urges, effectively dealing with stress and emotional triggers, learning from relapses, maintaining motivation, and finding meaning beyond smoking, individuals can overcome obstacles and embrace the freedom and health that comes with living smoke-free. Remember, each challenge you overcome brings you closer to a brighter, smoke-free future.

# Chapter 7: Embracing a Smoke-Free Future: Thriving in a Healthier Life

Introduction:

In this final chapter, we explore the profound impact of living a smoke-free life and the benefits it brings to overall health and well-being. We delve into the positive changes individuals can expect as they embrace their smoke-free future, providing inspiration and guidance for thriving in a healthier and more fulfilling life.

## Section 1: Physical Benefits of a Smoke-Free Life

Quitting smoking has immediate and long-term positive effects on physical health. We delve into the numerous benefits individuals can experience, such as improved lung function, reduced risk of cardiovascular disease, enhanced immunity, and increased energy levels. By understanding and appreciating these physical transformations, readers can find motivation and encouragement to continue their smoke-free journey.

## Section 2: Mental and Emotional Well-being

Smoking not only affects physical health but also takes a toll on mental and emotional well-being. We explore the positive impact of quitting smoking on mental health, including reduced anxiety and depression symptoms, improved mood, and enhanced self-esteem. By embracing a smoke-free life, individuals can experience greater emotional stability, increased clarity of mind, and a sense of empowerment.

Section 3: Financial Freedom: Saving Money and Achieving Goals

Smoking is not only detrimental to health but also a significant drain on finances. We discuss the financial benefits of quitting smoking, exploring the substantial savings individuals can accumulate over time. By redirecting the money previously spent on cigarettes towards meaningful goals, such as travel, education, or building a savings account, readers can embrace financial freedom and a sense of accomplishment.

Section 4: Improved Relationships and Social Interactions

Quitting smoking can positively impact personal relationships and social interactions. We delve into the ways in which a smoke-free lifestyle can enhance interpersonal connections, including the elimination of second-hand smoke exposure and the ability to engage more fully in social activities. By embracing a smoke-free future, individuals can strengthen relationships, foster healthier social connections, and enjoy a more vibrant social life.

Section 5: Inspiring Others: Becoming a Role Model

The journey to quitting smoking is not just a personal triumph but also an opportunity to inspire others. We explore the power of becoming a role model for family, friends, and even strangers who may be considering quitting smoking themselves. By sharing their own experiences and providing support and encouragement to others, readers can make a positive impact on the lives of those around them.

Section 6: Cultivating Self-Care and Wellness Practices

Living a smoke-free life opens up new opportunities for self-care and wellness practices. We discuss the importance of nurturing physical, mental, and emotional well-being through activities such as exercise, healthy eating, relaxation techniques, and mindfulness. By prioritizing self-care and embracing a holistic approach to wellness, readers can create a fulfilling and balanced life beyond smoking.

Conclusion:

As we conclude this chapter and our journey together, readers are encouraged to embrace their smoke-free future and the many benefits it brings. By experiencing improved physical health, enhanced mental and emotional well-being, financial freedom, enriched relationships, and the ability to inspire others, individuals can thrive in a healthier and more fulfilling life. Remember, your decision to quit smoking is not just a single event but a lifelong commitment to your well-being and the endless possibilities that lie ahead.

# Conclusion

Conclusion:

Congratulations on reaching the end of this book on quitting smoking and embracing a smoke-free life. Throughout the chapters, we have explored various aspects of the quitting process, providing insights, strategies, and inspiration to support your journey towards a healthier future. By making the decision to quit smoking, you have taken a significant step towards reclaiming control over your life and prioritizing your well-being.

Quitting smoking is not an easy task, and it requires determination, perseverance, and a willingness to embrace change. However, as you have learned, it is an immensely rewarding journey filled with countless benefits for your physical, mental, and emotional health.

Through the chapters, we discussed the importance of understanding the addiction, preparing for the quit day, adopting a smoke-free mindset, creating healthy habits, overcoming challenges, and ultimately thriving in a smoke-free life. You have gained valuable tools and insights to navigate triggers, manage cravings, find healthier coping mechanisms, and overcome setbacks.

Remember, quitting smoking is not a linear process. It may involve ups and downs, moments of strength and moments of weakness. What matters most is your commitment to yourself and your desire to live a healthier and smoke-free life. If you experience setbacks or relapses, don't be discouraged. Use those moments as opportunities for learning, growth, and renewed determination.

As you continue your smoke-free journey, embrace the positive changes that come with it. Celebrate milestones, both big and small, and acknowledge the progress you have made. Embrace the physical benefits of improved lung function, reduced health risks, and increased energy. Enjoy the freedom from the financial burden of smoking and the ability to redirect your resources towards your goals and aspirations.

Furthermore, relish in the enhanced relationships and social interactions that come with being smoke-free. Share your experience with others, become a source of inspiration and support, and make a difference in the lives of those around you. Cultivate self-care practices and prioritize your overall well-being, nurturing your mind, body, and spirit.

Remember, quitting smoking is a lifelong commitment, and the journey does not end here. Stay vigilant and continue to reinforce your smoke-free lifestyle. Surround yourself with a supportive network of friends, family, or support groups who understand and respect your decision. Seek help when needed and never hesitate to reach out for support.

As you move forward into your smoke-free future, always remember that you have the power to shape your life and create a healthier, happier, and more fulfilling existence. Embrace this newfound freedom and the countless opportunities that lie ahead. You have taken a significant step towards a brighter and smoke-free future, and with determination, perseverance, and the strategies you have learned, you can continue to thrive in your smoke-free life.

Congratulations once again, and may your journey be filled with joy, fulfillment, and abundant health.

www.ingramcontent.com/pod-product-compliance
Lightning Source LLC
Chambersburg PA
CBHW051713250726